PROSTATE CANCER PREVENTION COOKBOOK

Delicious Recipes for Prostate Cancer Prevention

Smart Desty

Copyright © 2023 by [Smart Desty]

This book is a work of nonfiction. While some of the names of people, places, and events have been changed, the author has made every effort to provide accurate information. The author and publisher are not responsible for any omissions or errors that may occur.

Table of Contents

INTRODUCTION

James was a middle-aged man who had been struggling with prostate cancer for several years. He had gone through several treatments and medications, but he was still not feeling well. He was having difficulty eating, and he was losing weight. He was becoming increasingly frustrated, as he felt like he was not making any progress.

One day, he saw a flyer for a new cookbook, called "Prostate Cancer Cookbook". He was intrigued and decided to give it a try.

When he opened the book, he was surprised to find that it was full of delicious recipes that were specifically tailored to help people with prostate cancer. He was amazed at how much thought and effort the authors had put into the book. The recipes were easy to prepare, and all of the ingredients were readily available at his local grocery store.

He decided to try some of the recipes, and he was pleasantly surprised. The food was delicious, and it was full of nutrients that he needed to help fight his cancer. He also noticed that he was feeling better after eating the food.

James followed the recipes in the cookbook for several weeks, and he noticed that he was starting to make progress in his fight against cancer. He was gradually gaining weight, and his energy levels were increasing. He was feeling better than he had in a long time.

The Prostate Cancer Cookbook had helped James in more ways than he ever thought possible. He was feeling better, and he was even starting to enjoy preparing meals again. He was thankful to have found this book, as it had helped him turn his life around.

Prostate cancer is a serious health issue that affects millions of men around the world. While treatment for prostate cancer can be difficult, there are many things that men can do to help manage their condition. One of the best ways to help manage prostate cancer is through diet. Eating a healthy, balanced diet can help to reduce the risk of developing prostate cancer, as well as help to manage its symptoms.

That's why we have put together this Prostate Cancer Cookbook. This cookbook is full of delicious and nutritious recipes specifically designed for men with prostate cancer. All of the recipes are low in saturated fat, sodium, and added sugar, and are high in fiber, vitamins, and minerals. They are also full of plant-based proteins, healthy fats, and antioxidants, which are all important for supporting the health of the prostate.

In addition to the recipes, this cookbook also includes helpful information about prostate cancer, such as information on diagnosis, treatments, and side effects. We hope that this cookbook will provide you with the tools and support you need to make healthy decisions about your diet and prostate health.

The Prostate Cancer Cookbook also includes a variety of tips and tricks for making cooking easier, from meal planning and preparation to shopping for the right ingredients. We also provide a list of recommended kitchen tools and appliances, so you can make sure you have everything you need to make your favorite recipes.

We hope that this cookbook will be a valuable resource to help you make healthy, delicious meals that are tailored to your specific dietary needs. With the right recipes and a bit of knowledge, you can make a difference in your prostate health. It's time to get cooking!

[14]

CHAPTER 1:

UNDERSTANDING PROSTATE CANCER

One type of cancer that affects the prostate, a gland in the male reproductive system, is prostate cancer. It is the most common type of cancer in men and the second most common cause of cancer death in men, behind lung cancer. Prostate cancer is often slow-growing, but can spread to other parts of the body if left untreated.

The cause of prostate cancer is not known, but some factors can increase a man's risk. These include age, family history, race, and lifestyle factors such as smoking and diet. Prostate cancer is most common in men over the age of 50, and is rare in men younger than 40. African-American men have the highest rate of prostate cancer, while Asian-American men have the lowest rate.

Prostate cancer is usually diagnosed through screening tests such as a digital rectal exam (DRE) or a prostate-specific antigen (PSA) blood test. If either of these tests is abnormal, further tests such as a biopsy and/or imaging scans may be ordered to confirm the diagnosis.

Treatments for prostate cancer vary and depend on the stage of the cancer, the patient's age and health, and other factors. Options include surgery, radiation therapy, hormone therapy, chemotherapy, immunotherapy, and active surveillance. Surgery is the most common treatment, and can include removal of the prostate (radical prostatectomy), or removal of just the tumor (partial or segmental prostatectomy). Radiation therapy involves the use of x-rays or other types of radiation to kill cancer cells. Hormone therapy is used to reduce androgen levels, which can slow or stop the growth of prostate cancer. Chemotherapy is usually used in combination with other treatments, and immunotherapy involves stimulating the body's immune system to fight cancer cells. Active surveillance, or watchful waiting, is an option for men with low-risk prostate cancer who are not candidates for other treatments.

The prognosis for prostate cancer depends on the stage of the cancer, the patient's age and health, and other factors. In general, the earlier prostate cancer is detected and treated, the better the prognosis. Prostate cancer can be cured if it is caught and treated early enough.

It is important for men to discuss prostate cancer screening with their doctor. Screening tests can detect prostate cancer early, when it is most treatable. Men should also be aware of the signs and symptoms of prostate cancer, which can include difficulty starting or stopping urination, weak or interrupted urine flow, frequent urination, and pain or burning during urination.

Prostate cancer can be a frightening diagnosis, but there are many treatments available that can lead to a successful outcome. By understanding prostate cancer and the risk factors associated with it, men can make informed decisions about their own health and the best treatment options for them.

CHAPTER 2: SYMPTOMS AND RISK FACTORS

The most prevalent type of cancer in American males is prostate cancer. It is estimated that one in nine men will be diagnosed with prostate cancer in their lifetime. The risk of developing prostate cancer increases with age and is more common in African American men. Prostate cancer is a serious disease that can be difficult to detect in its early stages. It is important to be aware of the symptoms and risk factors associated with prostate cancer so that it can be diagnosed and treated as soon as possible.

The most common symptom of prostate cancer is difficulty in urinating. This can include a weak or intermittent stream of urine, a sense of not being able to completely empty the bladder, or having to urinate frequently. Other symptoms may include blood in the urine or semen, pain in the back, hips, or thighs, and difficulty achieving or maintaining an erection.

There are several risk factors for developing prostate cancer. Age is among the most significant risk factors. The risk of developing prostate cancer increases with age, with most cases occurring in men over the age of 65. African American men are also at an increased risk for developing prostate cancer, with a risk that is more than twice that of white men.

Another significant risk factor for prostate cancer is family history. Men with a father or brother who have had prostate cancer have an increased risk of developing the disease. Other risk factors include obesity, smoking, and a sedentary lifestyle.

The exact cause of prostate cancer is unknown, but certain lifestyle choices can increase the risk of developing the disease. Eating a balanced diet that is low in red and processed meats and high in vegetables, fruits, and whole grains can help reduce the risk. Additionally, regular physical activity, maintaining a healthy weight, and avoiding smoking can help reduce the risk.

If prostate cancer is suspected, a doctor will typically order a prostate specific antigen (PSA) test to measure the levels of this protein in the blood. If the PSA level is higher than normal, a biopsy may be recommended to confirm the diagnosis.

In most cases, prostate cancer can be successfully treated if caught early. Treatments may include surgery, radiation therapy, hormone therapy, or chemotherapy. The type of treatment that is recommended depends on the stage and severity of the cancer.

Prostate cancer is a serious disease, but it can be successfully treated if caught early. Knowing the symptoms and risk factors associated with prostate cancer can help men take steps to reduce their risk and seek prompt medical attention if they experience any of the warning signs. It is important to talk to your doctor about any concerns or questions you may have about prostate cancer.

Lifestyle changes can also help reduce the risk of prostate cancer. Eating a healthy diet that includes plenty of fruits, vegetables, and whole grains, exercising regularly, and maintaining a healthy weight can all help reduce the risk. Additionally, avoiding smoking and excessive alcohol consumption can help reduce the risk.

Prostate cancer can be a difficult disease to detect in its early stages. However, if caught early, it can be successfully treated. Be sure to talk to your doctor about any symptoms you may be experiencing and discuss your risk factors for prostate cancer. It is important to take steps to reduce your risk and seek prompt medical attention if you experience any of the warning signs. With early diagnosis and treatment, prostate cancer can be successfully managed.

CHAPTER 3: DIAGNOSIS AND TREATMENT OPTIONS

Prostate cancer is a type of cancer that affects the prostate, a gland in the male reproductive system. It is the second most common type of cancer among men in the United States and is the fifth leading cause of death from cancer in men. Prostate cancer can be treated with surgery, radiation, hormone therapy, chemotherapy and/or other treatments, depending on the stage and type of cancer.

DIAGNOSIS

The diagnosis of prostate cancer usually begins with a physical examination, including a digital rectal exam (DRE) to feel for any abnormalities in the prostate, and a prostate-specific antigen (PSA) test to measure the level of PSA in the blood. Usually, if the result of the PSA test is elevated, it may indicate the presence of prostate cancer.

In addition to the physical exam and PSA test, a biopsy of the prostate may also be performed. During this procedure, a small sample of tissue is taken from the prostate and examined under a microscope. This helps to determine the presence and type of cancer, as well as the stage of the cancer.

TREATMENT OPTIONS

The treatment for prostate cancer depends on the stage of the cancer and the type of cancer.

Surgery

Surgery is often used to treat prostate cancer, especially if the cancer is localized and confined to the prostate. The main type of surgery used to treat prostate cancer is a radical prostatectomy, which involves removing the entire prostate gland, along with nearby tissues and lymph nodes. Other types of surgery may be used to treat advanced cases of prostate cancer, such as a pelvic lymph node dissection or a transurethral resection of the prostate.

Radiation

Radiation therapy may be used to treat localized prostate cancer or to relieve symptoms of advanced prostate cancer. There are two main types of radiation therapy used to treat prostate cancer, external beam radiation therapy (EBRT) and brachytherapy, which involves placing radioactive seeds into the prostate.

Hormone Therapy

Advanced prostate cancer is treated with hormone treatment. This type of therapy works by blocking the production of testosterone, a hormone that helps fuel the growth of prostate cancer cells. Commonly used drugs for hormone therapy include leuprolide, goserelin, and flutamide.

Chemotherapy

Chemotherapy is also used to treat advanced prostate cancer. This type of treatment involves using drugs to stop the growth of cancer cells. Common drugs used in chemotherapy include docetaxel, cabazitaxel, and estramustine.

Other Treatments

These include immunotherapy, which uses drugs to boost the body's immune system to fight the cancer, and targeted therapy, which uses drugs to target specific molecules in the cancer cells.

Prostate cancer is a serious disease that requires careful diagnosis and treatment. It is important to talk to your doctor about the best treatment options for your individual case. Depending on the stage and type of cancer, surgery, radiation, hormone therapy, chemotherapy, or other treatments may be used to treat the cancer. It is important to discuss all of the treatment options with your doctor and make sure you understand the risks and benefits of each option.

Other treatments that may be used to treat prostate cancer include cryotherapy, which uses extreme cold to destroy cancer cells, and high-intensity focused ultrasound (HIFU), which uses sound waves to target and destroy cancer cells. Other treatments such as photodynamic therapy and brachytherapy may also be used to treat localized prostate cancer.

In addition to the treatments mentioned above, there are many other therapies that may be used to treat prostate cancer. These include lifestyle changes such as quitting smoking, eating a healthy diet, and exercising regularly. complementary treatments including yoga, acupuncture, and massage may also be used to help manage symptoms and side effects of prostate cancer treatments. It is important to discuss all of these therapies with your doctor before beginning any treatment.

Prostate cancer is a serious condition that requires careful diagnosis and treatment. Treatment options vary depending on the stage and type of cancer, so it is important to talk to your doctor about the best treatment plan for your individual case. With proper diagnosis and treatment, many men with prostate cancer can live long, healthy lives.

CHAPTER 4: NUTRITION AND PROSTATE CANCER

Prostate cancer is one of the most common types of cancer in men, and it is generally caused by a combination of genetics, lifestyle, and environmental factors. One of the most important ways to help reduce your risk of prostate cancer is to maintain a healthy lifestyle, and this includes eating a nutritious diet. Nutrition plays a key role in reducing the risk of prostate cancer, as well as helping to manage and even prevent it.

A healthy diet is one that is low in saturated and trans fats, and high in fiber, fruits, vegetables, and whole grains. Fruits and vegetables are packed with phytochemicals, which are powerful antioxidants that can help protect against cancer. Eating a diet rich in fruits and vegetables may reduce the risk of prostate cancer by up to 25%. Whole grains such as oatmeal, brown rice, and barley are also important for prostate health, as they contain high levels of fiber and other important vitamins and minerals. Eating at least five servings of fruits and vegetables every day is recommended for optimal health.

In addition to eating a healthy diet, reducing your intake of red and processed meats can also help reduce your risk of prostate cancer. Red meats such as beef, pork, and lamb are high in saturated and trans fats, which can increase your risk of developing cancer. Processed meats, such as hot dogs and deli meats, are also high in saturated and trans fats and are linked to an increased risk of prostate cancer. Limit your intake of red and processed meats to no more than 18 ounces per week.

Another important factor in reducing your risk of prostate cancer is to maintain a healthy weight.

Being overweight or obese can increase your risk of prostate cancer, so it's important to follow a healthy diet and exercise regularly. Eating a diet that is high in fiber, fruits, vegetables, and whole grains, and limiting your intake of saturated and trans fats can help you maintain a healthy weight. Additionally, regular exercise can help you reduce your risk of prostate cancer and manage your weight.

Getting enough vitamin D from the sun or from dietary sources can also help reduce your risk of prostate cancer. Vitamin D helps your body absorb calcium, which is important for maintaining healthy bones. Additionally, studies have shown that vitamin D can help reduce the risk of prostate cancer by up to 20%. The best sources of vitamin D are fortified dairy products, fatty fish like tuna and salmon, and sunlight.

A nutritious diet is an important part of reducing the risk of prostate cancer. Eating a diet that is low in saturated and trans fats and high in fiber, fruits, vegetables, and whole grains can help reduce your risk of prostate cancer. Additionally, reducing your intake of red and processed meats and maintaining a healthy weight can help reduce your risk of prostate cancer. Finally, getting enough vitamin D can also help reduce your risk of prostate cancer. Eating a nutritious diet and following a healthy lifestyle can help you reduce your risk of prostate cancer and improve your overall health.

In addition to eating a nutritious diet and maintaining a healthy lifestyle, there are other things you can do to reduce your risk of prostate cancer. Avoiding tobacco use and limiting alcohol consumption can help reduce your risk of prostate cancer. Additionally, getting regular check-ups with your doctor can help detect prostate cancer early, when it is most treatable. Finally, there are some supplements that may help reduce the risk of prostate cancer, such as lycopene, selenium, and omega-3 fatty acids. Find out from your doctor which supplements can be helpful for you.

Eating a nutritious diet and following a healthy lifestyle can help reduce your risk of prostate cancer and improve your overall health. If you are at a higher risk of prostate cancer, talk to your doctor about further steps you can take to reduce your risk. Developing healthy habits now can help you stay healthy and reduce your risk of prostate cancer in the future.

[36]

CHAPTER 5: EXERCISE AND PROSTATE CANCER

Prostate cancer is a serious health issue that affects many men around the world. While the exact cause of prostate cancer is still unknown, there is evidence to suggest that exercise may play a role in helping to reduce the risk of developing this type of cancer. In this article, we will explore the impact of exercise on prostate cancer, the types of exercises that may be beneficial, and the ways in which men can reduce their risk of developing this disease.

Exercise is a type of physical activity that can help to reduce the risk of a variety of health conditions, including prostate cancer. Exercise helps to reduce inflammation, which can help to reduce the risk of developing cancer. Additionally, exercise has been linked to a decrease in circulating testosterone, which can reduce the risk of prostate cancer. Furthermore, exercise can help to reduce weight, which can also reduce the risk of prostate cancer.

There are various types of exercise that have been linked to a reduction in prostate cancer risk. Cardiovascular exercise, such as running, cycling, or swimming, can help to reduce inflammation and aid in weight loss. Resistance training, such as weightlifting, can also be beneficial in reducing the risk of prostate cancer, as it is linked to an increase in testosterone, which can help to reduce the risk of prostate cancer. Additionally, yoga and stretching exercises can help to reduce stress, which can also reduce the risk of developing prostate cancer.

In addition to exercise, there are other lifestyle changes that men can make to reduce their risk of developing prostate cancer. Eating a healthy diet is one of the best ways to reduce the risk of prostate cancer, as it helps to reduce inflammation and maintain a healthy weight. Additionally, quitting smoking and limiting alcohol consumption can help to reduce the risk of prostate cancer. Furthermore, men should try to get regular check-ups with their doctor to ensure that any potential issues are caught and treated as soon as possible.

Exercise can play an important role in reducing the risk of developing prostate cancer. Exercise helps to reduce inflammation, reduce circulating testosterone, and aid in weight loss. Additionally, there are other lifestyle changes that men can make to reduce their risk of developing this disease, such as eating a healthy diet, quitting smoking, and limiting alcohol consumption. Lastly, Regular check-ups with a doctor can help to ensure that any potential issues are caught and treated as soon as possible.

Prostate cancer is a serious health issue that affects many men around the world, and while the exact cause of this type of cancer is still unknown, there is evidence to suggest that exercise may play a role in helping to reduce the risk of developing this type of cancer. Exercise is a type of physical activity that can help to reduce the risk of a variety of health conditions, including prostate cancer. Exercise helps to reduce inflammation, which can help to reduce the risk of developing cancer. Additionally, exercise can help to reduce weight, which can also reduce the risk of prostate cancer. There are various types of exercise that have been linked to a reduction in prostate cancer risk, such as cardiovascular exercise, resistance training, stretching and yoga.

Cardiovascular exercise, such as running, cycling, or swimming, can help to reduce inflammation and aid in weight loss. Resistance training, such as weightlifting, can also be beneficial in reducing the risk of prostate cancer, as it is linked to an increase in testosterone, which can help to reduce the risk of prostate cancer. Additionally, yoga and stretching exercises can help to reduce stress, which can also reduce the risk of developing prostate cancer.

In addition to exercise, there are other lifestyle changes that men can make to reduce their risk of developing prostate cancer. Eating a healthy diet is one of the best ways to reduce the risk of prostate cancer, as it helps to reduce inflammation and maintain a healthy weight. Additionally, quitting smoking and limiting alcohol consumption can help to reduce the risk of prostate cancer. Furthermore, men should try to get regular check-ups with their doctor to ensure that any potential issues are caught and treated as soon as possible.

Regular physical activity is important for overall health and can also help to reduce the risk of prostate cancer. Exercise can take many forms, such as walking, running, biking, swimming, and weightlifting. When engaging in exercise, it is important to start slowly and build up to more vigorous activities over time. Additionally, it is important to listen to your body and stop if you experience any pain or discomfort.

It is also important to stay hydrated when engaging in physical activity, as dehydration can lead to fatigue and other health issues. Additionally, it is important to get enough rest in between exercise sessions to give your body time to rest and recover. It is important to wear appropriate clothing and footwear when exercising to reduce the risk of injury.

Exercise can play an important role in reducing the risk of developing prostate cancer. Exercise helps to reduce inflammation, reduce circulating testosterone, and aid in weight loss. Additionally, there are other lifestyle changes that men can make to reduce their risk of developing this disease, such as eating a healthy diet, quitting smoking, and limiting alcohol consumption. Lastly, Regular check-ups with a doctor can help to ensure that any potential issues are caught and treated as soon as possible. By taking these steps, men can reduce their risk of developing prostate cancer and improve their overall health.

CHAPTER 5: TREATMENT OPTIONS FOR PROSTATE CANCER

Prostate cancer is one of the most common cancers in men, and there are a variety of treatment options available for those who have been diagnosed with it. Treatment for prostate cancer will vary depending on the stage and grade of the cancer, as well as the overall health of the patient. Some treatments are standard and recommended for all prostate cancer patients, while others may be more specialized or tailored to the individual patient.

Surgery

Surgery is one of the most common treatments for prostate cancer. The type of surgery will depend on the stage and grade of the cancer, as well as the overall health of the patient. Generally, prostatectomy is the most common type of surgery used to treat prostate cancer. This procedure involves the removal of the entire prostate gland and some of the surrounding tissue. There are several types of prostatectomy, including open, laparoscopic, and robotic surgery. Depending on the stage of cancer, the surgeon may also remove nearby lymph nodes.

Radiation Therapy

This treatment uses high-energy X-rays or other types of radiation to kill cancer cells. Radiation therapy can be used as the sole treatment for prostate cancer or it can be used in conjunction with other treatments, such as surgery or hormone therapy.

The most used form of radiation therapy is external beam radiation therapy. This involves a beam of radiation being aimed at the prostate from outside the body. Intensity-modulated radiation therapy is a newer type of external beam radiation therapy that allows for a more precise dose of radiation to be delivered to the cancerous area.

Brachytherapy is another type of radiation therapy. This involves placing tiny radioactive pellets directly into the prostate gland. Brachytherapy can be done in conjunction with external beam radiation therapy.

Hormone Therapy

Hormone therapy is used to reduce the levels of testosterone in the body. Testosterone is an important hormone in men and helps to stimulate the growth of prostate cancer cells. By reducing the levels of testosterone in the body, it can help to slow down or stop the growth of prostate cancer cells.

Hormone therapy can be used as the sole treatment for prostate cancer or it can be used in combination with other treatments, such as surgery or radiation therapy. The most common hormone therapy used is an LHRH (Luteinizing Hormone Releasing Hormone) agonist. This type of therapy works by blocking the release of testosterone from the testes. Another type of hormone therapy is an anti-androgen. This type of therapy works by blocking the effects of testosterone on prostate cancer cells.

Chemotherapy

Chemotherapy is a treatment option for prostate cancer that involves the use of drugs to kill cancer cells. Chemotherapy can be used as a primary treatment for prostate cancer or it can be used in combination with other treatments. Generally, chemotherapy is used for advanced prostate cancer that has spread beyond the prostate gland.

Immunotherapy

Immunotherapy is a newer treatment option for prostate cancer. This treatment uses medications or other substances to stimulate the body's own immune system to fight the cancer cells. Immunotherapy can be used as a primary treatment or it can be used in combination with other treatments.

Clinical Trials

Clinical trials are research studies that explore new treatments or new ways of using existing treatments. These trials are conducted to determine if a certain treatment is safe and effective. Clinical trials are available for all stages of prostate cancer. These trials can offer access to treatments that are not yet widely available.

No matter which treatment option is chosen, it is important to have a good understanding of the risks and benefits associated with each treatment. It is also important to talk to your doctor about all of the available treatment options, so that you can make an informed decision about which treatment is best for you.

CHAPTER 7: INTEGRATIVE MEDICINE AND PROSTATE CANCER

Integrative medicine is a holistic approach to healthcare that combines traditional medicine, alternative, and complementary medicine. It is based on the belief that the body, mind, and spirit must be in balance to achieve optimum health. Integrative medicine involves a range of therapies and treatments, including lifestyle and dietary changes, stress-management techniques, physical activity, and mind-body therapies.

In the case of prostate cancer, integrative medicine can be used to support conventional treatments, such as surgery and radiation therapy. Integrative medicine can also be used as a complementary therapy for those who are looking for additional ways to support their health and wellbeing. There is a range of integrative treatments available, such as nutrition and herbal therapies, acupuncture, yoga, meditation, and massage.

Nutrition and herbal therapies are a cornerstone of integrative medicine. Eating a healthy and balanced diet is essential for the prevention and management of prostate cancer. A diet rich in fruits and vegetables, whole grains, lean proteins, healthy fats, and low in processed foods is recommended. Additionally, certain herbs and supplements can be used to support the body's natural healing processes and may help to reduce the risk of prostate cancer.

Acupuncture is another popular form of integrative medicine. Acupuncture is an ancient Chinese healing technique that involves the insertion of fine needles into specific points on the body. It is believed that this stimulates the body's natural healing responses, and may be beneficial in reducing symptoms of prostate cancer and in some cases, improving the quality of life of patients.

Yoga and meditation are also integral parts of integrative medicine. Yoga can help to reduce stress and anxiety, improve sleep, and support overall physical and mental health. Meditation can also help to reduce stress and anxiety, as well as improve focus and mental clarity.

Massage is a form of integrative medicine that can help to reduce stress, improve circulation, and promote relaxation. Massage therapy can be used by prostate cancer patients to help reduce fatigue, pain, and other symptoms associated with the disease.

Integrative medicine can be beneficial in the treatment and management of prostate cancer. It can help to reduce symptoms, improve quality of life, and support overall health and wellbeing. It is important to discuss your options with your doctor before starting any integrative therapy.

CHAPTER 8: PROSTATE CANCER SUPPORT GROUPS

Prostate cancer is a serious and potentially life-threatening disease that affects many men in the United States and throughout the world. It is the second most common form of cancer among men, and the third most common cause of death from cancer in the United States. The good news is that with early detection and improved treatments, many men now survive prostate cancer. However, the diagnosis of prostate cancer can be a difficult and stressful experience, and many men find it helpful to join a prostate cancer support group to help them cope with the diagnosis and treatment.

Prostate cancer support groups are typically made up of a group of men who have been diagnosed with prostate cancer and their family members. These groups provide support, information and understanding for those affected by prostate cancer. They provide a safe and confidential environment for members to discuss their concerns, fears, and feelings about their diagnosis and treatment.

Members of prostate cancer support groups often find that the group can provide a sense of community and comfort. Members can discuss the physical and emotional effects of prostate cancer and learn from one another. They can also receive practical advice and support from other men who have been through the same experience.

In addition to providing emotional and practical support, prostate cancer support groups can also provide educational information on prostate cancer, including the latest developments in treatments and research. This can be especially beneficial for men who are newly diagnosed, as they can gain access to information and resources that may not be available to them through their doctors.

Prostate cancer support groups can also provide access to resources such as patient advocacy groups, financial assistance programs, and local support groups. These resources can be invaluable for men and their families who are struggling to cope with the diagnosis and treatment of prostate cancer.

Prostate cancer support groups offer a sense of hope and optimism for members. They provide a place for members to talk about their experiences and to receive encouragement from others in similar situations. This can be especially beneficial for men who are feeling isolated and overwhelmed by the diagnosis and treatment of prostate cancer.

Prostate cancer support groups can be a beneficial resource for men who have been diagnosed with prostate cancer. They provide a safe, confidential environment for members to discuss their concerns and feelings, as well as access to information and resources. They also offer a sense of community and hope for members, which can be invaluable during such a difficult time. For these reasons, many men find that joining a prostate cancer support group can be a beneficial and helpful experience.

CHAPTER 9: HEALTHY RECIPES PROSTATE CANCER PREVENTION

Twenty (20) Breakfast Recipes

1. Protein-Packed Overnight Oats: Pre-soak ½ cup of rolled oats in ½ cup of almond milk overnight. In the morning, top with ½ cup of blueberries, ½ cup of walnuts, and a scoop of protein powder. Preparation: 5 minutes;

2. Avocado Toast: Mash ½ an avocado and spread on a whole wheat toast. Top with a sprinkle of red pepper flakes, a squeeze of lemon juice, and a dash of Himalayan sea salt. Preparation time: 5 minutes;

3. Chia Seed Pudding: Mix together ½ cup of chia seeds with 1 cup of almond milk and a teaspoon of honey. Let sit for 10 minutes and top with your favorite berries. Prep time: 10 minutes; Total time: 20 minutes.

4. Veggie Omelet: Beat together two eggs with a pinch of salt and pepper and pour into a pan. Add in ½ cup of diced bell peppers and ¼ cup of chopped spinach and cook until the eggs are set. Prep time: 5 minutes; Total time: 10 minutes.

5. Kale and Quinoa Bowl: Cook ½ cup of quinoa according to package instructions and mix with 1 cup of kale that has been sautéed in olive oil. Olive oil and Parmesan cheese should be drizzled on top. Preparation time: 10 minutes

6. Smoked Salmon and Avocado Toast: Top a slice of whole wheat toast with smoked salmon, mashed avocado, and a sprinkle of capers. Drizzle with olive oil and lemon juice. Preparation: 5 minutes;

7. Greek Yogurt Parfait: Layer ½ cup of Greek yogurt with ½ cup of berries, walnuts, and a drizzle of honey. Prep time: 5 minutes; Total time: 10 minutes.

8. Tomato and Mozzarella Salad: Slice a tomato and top with fresh mozzarella cheese, a sprinkle of salt and pepper, and a drizzle of olive oil. Prep time: 5 minutes; Total time: 10 minutes.

9. Hard-Boiled Egg: Boil a pot of water and add in one or two eggs. Cook for 8 minutes and serve with a sprinkle of salt and pepper. Prep time: 5 minutes; Total time: 10 minutes.

10. Fruit and Nut Smoothie: Blend together ½ cup of almond milk, ½ cup of frozen berries, and a handful of your favorite nuts. Prep time: 5 minutes; Total time: 10 minutes.

11. Quinoa Porridge: Cook ½ cup of quinoa according to package instructions and add to a pot of boiling water. Cook until the quinoa is creamy and stir in a tablespoon of honey and a handful of your favorite nuts. Prep time: 5 minutes; Total time: 10 minutes.

12. Avocado Toast with Egg: Top a slice of whole wheat toast with mashed avocado and a sunny side up egg. Sprinkle with a pinch of salt and pepper. Prep time: 5 minutes; Total time: 10 minutes.

13. Spinach and Mushroom Frittata: Beat together four eggs with a pinch of salt and pepper and pour into a pan. Add in ½ cup of diced mushrooms, ½ cup of spinach, and a handful of Parmesan cheese. Cook until the eggs are set. Prep time: 5 minutes; Total time: 10 minutes.

14. Chia Seed Pudding with Nuts and Seeds: Mix together ½ cup of chia seeds with 1 cup of almond milk and a teaspoon of honey. Let sit for 10 minutes and top with your favorite nuts and seeds. Prep time: 10 minutes; Total time: 20 minutes.

15. Whole Wheat Pancakes: Whisk together 1 cup of whole wheat flour, 1 teaspoon of baking powder, 1 tablespoon of honey, and 1 cup of almond milk. Cook on a hot pan for 2-3 minutes per side. Prep time: 5 minutes; Total time: 10 minutes.

16. Fruit and Nut Oatmeal: Cook ½ cup of oats according to package instructions and top with your favorite berries, nuts, and a drizzle of honey. Prep time: 5 minutes; Total time: 10 minutes.

17. Veggie and Cheese Burrito: Heat a whole wheat tortilla in a pan and top with ½ cup of diced bell peppers, ¼ cup of chopped spinach, ¼ cup of shredded cheese, and a pinch of salt and pepper. Wrap and enjoy. Prep time: 5 minutes; Total time: 10 minutes.

18. Greek Yogurt Bowl: Top ½ cup of Greek yogurt with ½ cup of berries, ½ cup of walnuts, and a drizzle of honey. Prep time: 5 minutes; Total time: 10 minutes.

19. Baked Sweet Potato: Pierce a sweet potato with a fork and bake in a preheated oven for 40 minutes. Top with a sprinkle of cinnamon and a drizzle of honey. Prep time: 5 minutes; Total time: 45 minutes.

20. Banana and Almond Butter Toast: Toast a slice of whole wheat toast and top with mashed banana and almond butter. Sprinkle with a pinch of cinnamon and a drizzle of honey. Prep time: 5 minutes; Total time: 10 minutes.

Lunch Recipes

1. Mediterranean Lentil Salad: Cook 2 cups of lentils according to package instructions. Once cooled, add in 1 cup of diced tomatoes, 1/2 cup of diced cucumber, 1/2 cup of diced red onion, 1/2 cup of diced bell pepper, 2 tablespoons of olive oil, 2 tablespoons of red wine vinegar, 1/2 teaspoon of garlic powder, 1/2 teaspoon of paprika, 1/2 teaspoon of dried oregano, and salt and pepper to taste. Mix together and serve. Prep Time: 15 minutes.

2. Spicy Chili: Heat 2 tablespoons of olive oil in a large pot over medium heat. Add in 1 diced onion, 1 diced bell pepper, 2 cloves of minced garlic, 1 teaspoon of chili powder, 1 teaspoon of smoked paprika, 1/4 teaspoon of cumin, and 1/4 teaspoon of oregano. Cook for 5 minutes, stirring occasionally. Pour in 1 can of diced tomatoes, 1 can of black beans, 1 can of kidney beans, 1 can of corn, and 1 cup of vegetable broth. Simmer for 20 minutes. Add salt and pepper to taste. Serve. Prep Time: 20 minutes.

3. Lentil Burger: In a food processor, combine 1 cup of cooked lentils, 1/2 cup of cooked quinoa, 1/2 cup of oat flour, 1/4 cup of diced onion, 1/4 cup of diced bell pepper, 1/4 cup of diced mushrooms, 1 teaspoon of garlic powder, 1 teaspoon of dried oregano, 1 teaspoon of smoked paprika, and salt and pepper to taste. Pulse until combined. Form into 4 patties. Heat a large skillet over medium heat. Add the patties and cook for 4 minutes on each side. Serve. Prep Time: 15 minutes.

4. Eggplant Parmesan: Preheat oven to 400 degrees F. Slice 1 large eggplant into 1/4-inch slices. Sprinkle with salt and let sit for 10 minutes.

Pat dry. Brush with 1/4 cup of olive oil. Place on a baking sheet and bake for 15 minutes. In a shallow bowl, combine 1/2 cup of bread crumbs, 1/4 cup of grated Parmesan cheese, 1 teaspoon of garlic powder, 1 teaspoon of dried oregano, 1 teaspoon of smoked paprika, and salt and pepper to taste. Dip the eggplant slices in the breadcrumb mixture and place back on the baking sheet. Bake for an additional 15 minutes. Serve. Prep Time: 25 minutes.

5. Roasted Beet Salad: Preheat oven to 425 degrees F. Wash and cut 4 beets into cubes. Place on a baking sheet and toss with 2 tablespoons of olive oil, 1 teaspoon of garlic powder, 1 teaspoon of dried oregano, 1 teaspoon of smoked paprika, and salt and pepper to taste. Roast for 20 minutes. Place the roasted beets in a large bowl and add in 1/4 cup of diced red onion, 1/4 cup of diced feta cheese, 1/4 cup of chopped walnuts, 2 tablespoons of olive oil, 2 tablespoons of red wine vinegar, and salt and pepper to taste. Mix together and serve. Prep Time: 25 minutes.

6. Cauliflower Rice Bowl: Heat a large skillet over medium heat. Add 1 tablespoon of olive oil, 1 teaspoon of garlic powder, 1 teaspoon of smoked paprika, 1/2 teaspoon of cumin, and salt and pepper to taste. Cook for 1 minute. Add 1 head of cauliflower that has been cut into florets and cook for an additional 5 minutes. Add 1/2 cup of diced bell peppers, 1/2 cup of diced tomatoes, and 1/4 cup of diced red onion. Cook for an additional 5 minutes. Serve. Prep Time: 10 minutes.

7. Zucchini Fritters: In a large bowl, combine 2 cups of grated zucchini, 1/4 cup of diced onion, 1/4 cup of diced bell pepper, 1/4 cup of chopped fresh parsley, 2 tablespoons of oat flour, 1 teaspoon of garlic powder, 1 teaspoon of smoked paprika, and salt and pepper to taste. Form into 8 patties and place on a baking sheet. Bake at 375 degrees F for 20 minutes. Serve. Prep Time: 25 minutes.

8. Quinoa and Black Bean Burrito: Heat a large skillet over medium heat. Add 2 tablespoons of olive oil, 1 teaspoon of garlic powder, 1 teaspoon of smoked paprika, 1/2 teaspoon of cumin, and salt and pepper to taste. Cook for 1 minute. Add 1 cup of cooked quinoa, 1 can of black beans, 1/4 cup of diced tomatoes, and 1/4 cup of diced onion. Cook for an additional 5 minutes. Serve in a whole wheat tortilla with your favorite salsa and guacamole. Prep Time: 10 minutes.

9. Sweet Potato Curry: Heat a large pot over medium heat. Add 2 tablespoons of olive oil, 1 teaspoon of garlic powder, 1 teaspoon of smoked paprika, 1 teaspoon of curry powder, and salt and pepper to taste. Cook for 1 minute. Add 1 diced onion, 1 diced bell pepper, 1 diced sweet potato, and 1 cup of vegetable broth. Simmer for 15 minutes. Add 1 can of coconut milk and 1 cup of cooked lentils. Simmer for an additional 10 minutes. Serve. Prep Time: 25 minutes.

10. Mediterranean Quinoa Bowl: Heat a large skillet over medium heat. Add 2 tablespoons of olive oil, 1 teaspoon of garlic powder, 1 teaspoon of smoked paprika, 1/2 teaspoon of oregano, and salt and pepper to taste. Cook for 1 minute. Add 1 cup of cooked quinoa, 1/4 cup of diced tomatoes, 1/4 cup of diced cucumber, 1/4 cup of diced red onion, 1/4 cup of diced olives, and 1/4 cup of crumbled feta cheese. Cook for an additional 5 minutes. Serve. Prep Time: 10 minutes.

11. Avocado Toast: Toast 2 slices of whole wheat bread. Mash 1/2 of an avocado and spread onto toast. Top with 1/4 cup of diced tomatoes, 1/4 cup of diced red onion, 1/4 teaspoon of garlic powder, 1/4 teaspoon of smoked paprika, and salt and pepper to taste. Serve. Prep Time: 5 minutes.

12. Baked Salmon: Preheat oven to 400 degrees F. Place 1 pound of salmon onto a baking sheet. Top with 2 tablespoons of olive oil, 1 teaspoon of garlic powder, 1 teaspoon of smoked paprika, 1 teaspoon of dried oregano, and salt and pepper to taste. Bake for 15 minutes. Serve. Prep Time: 5 minutes.

13. Roasted Vegetable Pasta: Preheat oven to 425 degrees F. Toss 1 head of cauliflower, 1 red bell pepper, and 1 yellow bell pepper with 2 tablespoons of olive oil, 1 teaspoon of garlic powder, 1 teaspoon of smoked paprika, and salt and pepper to taste. Place on a baking sheet and bake for 20 minutes. Meanwhile, cook 8 ounces of whole wheat pasta according to package instructions. Once the vegetables are done, add to the cooked pasta along with 1/4 cup of diced olives, 1/4 cup of crumbled feta cheese, and 2 tablespoons of olive oil. Mix together and serve. Prep Time: 25 minutes.

14. Grilled Chicken Skewers: Preheat grill to medium heat. In a large bowl, combine 2 tablespoons of olive oil, 1 teaspoon of garlic powder, 1 teaspoon of smoked paprika, 1/2 teaspoon of cumin, and salt and pepper to taste. Toss 1 pound of cubed chicken in the marinade. Thread onto 4 skewers and place on the grill. Grill for 10 minutes, flipping halfway through. Serve. Prep Time: 10 minutes.

15. Vegetable Stir Fry: Heat 1 tablespoon of olive oil in a large skillet over medium heat. Add 1 diced onion, 1 diced bell pepper, 1 diced zucchini, 1 diced carrot, 1/2 cup of diced mushrooms, 1 teaspoon of garlic powder, 1 teaspoon of smoked paprika, and salt and pepper to taste. Cook for 5 minutes, stirring occasionally. Add 1/4 cup of vegetable broth and 1/4 cup of peanut sauce. Cook for an additional 5 minutes. Serve. Prep Time: 10 minutes.

16. Stuffed Peppers: Preheat oven to 375 degrees F. In a large bowl, combine 1 cup of cooked quinoa, 1 can of black beans, 1/4 cup of diced tomatoes, 1/4 cup of diced onion, 1/4 cup of diced bell pepper, 1 teaspoon of garlic powder, 1 teaspoon of smoked paprika, and salt and pepper to taste. Mix together. Cut 4 bell peppers in half and remove the seeds. Stuff each pepper with the quinoa mixture and place on a baking sheet. Bake for 20 minutes. Serve. Prep Time: 25 minutes.

17. Cauliflower Rice Burrito Bowl: Heat a large skillet over medium heat. Add 1 tablespoon of olive oil, 1 teaspoon of garlic powder, 1 teaspoon of smoked paprika, and salt and pepper to taste. Cook for 1 minute. Add 1 head of cauliflower that has been cut into florets and cook for an additional 5 minutes. Add 1/2 cup of diced bell peppers, 1/2 cup of diced tomatoes, and 1/4 cup of diced red onion. Cook for an additional 5 minutes. Serve in a bowl with your favorite salsa, guacamole, and black beans. Prep Time: 10 minutes.

18. Chickpea and Spinach Salad: In a large bowl, combine 1 can of chickpeas, 2 cups of fresh baby spinach, 1/4 cup of diced red onion, 1/4 cup of diced tomatoes, 1/4 cup of diced cucumber, 2 tablespoons of olive oil, 2 tablespoons of red wine vinegar, 1 teaspoon of garlic powder, 1 teaspoon of smoked paprika, and salt and pepper to taste. Mix together and serve. Prep Time: 5 minutes.

19. Grilled Eggplant: Preheat grill to medium heat. Slice 1 large eggplant into 1/4-inch slices. Brush with 1/4 cup of olive oil and season with 1 teaspoon of garlic powder, 1 teaspoon of smoked paprika, and salt and pepper to taste. Grill for 10 minutes, flipping halfway through. Serve. Prep Time: 10 minutes.

20. Quinoa Bowl with Avocado and Corn: Heat a large skillet over medium heat. Add 2 tablespoons of olive oil, 1 teaspoon of garlic powder, 1 teaspoon of smoked paprika, and salt and pepper to taste. Cook for 1 minute. Add 1 cup of cooked quinoa, 1/4 cup of diced tomatoes, 1/4 cup of diced red onion, 1/4 cup of cooked corn, 1/4 cup of diced avocado, and 2 tablespoons of lime juice. Cook for an additional 5 minutes. Serve. Prep Time: 10 minutes.

Seventeen (17) Dinner recipes for Prostate Cancer prevention with prep time and instructions

1. Vegetable and Quinoa Bowl: In a medium saucepan, bring 1 cup quinoa and 2 cups vegetable broth to a boil. Reduce the heat and simmer for about 15 minutes or until the liquid is absorbed. Meanwhile, heat 1 tablespoon olive oil in a large skillet over medium-high heat. Add 2 cloves minced garlic and 1 chopped onion, and sauté for 3 minutes. Add 1 red bell pepper, 1/2 teaspoon dried oregano, and 1/4 teaspoon salt, stirring occasionally until the vegetables are tender. Fluff the quinoa with a fork, then stir in the sautéed vegetables. Serve with a sprinkle of feta cheese, if desired. Prep time: 20 minutes.

2. Roasted Salmon with Asparagus: Preheat oven to 425°F. Line a baking sheet with parchment paper and spray with cooking spray. Place 1 pound of fresh asparagus in the center of the baking sheet, leaving a small space for the salmon. Drizzle with 1 tablespoon of olive oil and season with salt and pepper. Place 2 (4-ounce) salmon filets on top of the asparagus. Squeeze juice of 1/2 lemon over the salmon, then sprinkle with 1 teaspoon of dried dill. Roast for 12-15 minutes or until the salmon is cooked through. Prep time: 10 minutes.

3. Baked Sweet Potatoes with Salmon: Preheat oven to 375°F. Line a baking sheet with parchment paper. Place 2 (4-ounce) salmon filets in the center of the baking sheet. Drizzle with 1 tablespoon of olive oil and season with 1/2 teaspoon of salt and pepper. Bake for 12-15 minutes or until the salmon is cooked through. Meanwhile, pierce 4 sweet potatoes with a fork and microwave for 8 minutes until softened. Cut the potatoes in half and place them on the baking sheet. Drizzle with olive oil and season with salt and pepper. Bake for an additional 15 minutes or until the sweet potatoes are golden brown and crispy. Serve the salmon and sweet potatoes together. Prep time: 20 minutes.

4. Grilled Chicken and Veggie Skewers: In a bowl, combine 1/4 cup olive oil, 1 teaspoon garlic powder, 1 teaspoon dried oregano, 1 teaspoon dried basil, 1/4 teaspoon salt, and 1/4 teaspoon freshly ground black pepper. Cut 2 boneless skinless chicken breasts into 1-inch cubes and add to the marinade. Let the chicken marinate for at least 30 minutes. Preheat an outdoor grill or indoor grill pan to medium-high heat. Meanwhile, cut a variety of vegetables into 1-inch cubes. You can use bell peppers, onions, zucchini, mushrooms, and cherry tomatoes. Thread the marinated chicken and vegetables onto metal skewers. Cook on the grill until the chicken is cooked through and the vegetables are lightly charred and tender, about 8-10 minutes, flipping once halfway through. Serve with your favorite side dish. Prep time: 40 minutes.

5. Lentil Soup: Heat 1 tablespoon of olive oil in a large pot over medium-high heat. Add 1 chopped onion and 2 cloves minced garlic and sauté for 3 minutes. Add 4 cups vegetable broth, 1 cup green lentils, 1 chopped carrot, 1/2 teaspoon dried oregano, 1/2 teaspoon dried thyme, 1 bay leaf, and 1/4 teaspoon salt. Bring to a boil, then reduce the heat and simmer for 25-30 minutes or until the lentils are tender. Remove from the heat and discard the bay leaf. Serve with a sprinkle of freshly chopped parsley, if desired. Prep time: 30 minutes.

6. Chickpea Curry: Heat 1 tablespoon of olive oil in a large pot over medium-high heat. Add 1 chopped onion, 2 cloves minced garlic, 1 teaspoon freshly grated ginger, 1 teaspoon ground cumin, 1 teaspoon ground coriander, 1/2 teaspoon ground turmeric, and 1/4 teaspoon cayenne pepper. Sauté for 3 minutes. Add 1 can of diced tomatoes and 1 can of chickpeas and stir until combined. Simmer for 10 minutes. Serve over cooked brown rice. Prep time: 15 minutes.

7. Eggplant Parmesan: Preheat oven to 375°F. Place 1/2 cup of breadcrumbs, 1/2 cup of freshly grated Parmesan cheese, and 1/4 teaspoon of garlic powder in a shallow bowl and set aside. Slice 1 large eggplant into 1/4-inch thick slices. Dip each slice into a bowl of beaten egg, then into the breadcrumb mixture. Place the slices on a baking sheet lined with parchment paper and bake for 15 minutes or until the eggplant is golden brown. Meanwhile, heat 1 tablespoon of olive oil in a medium saucepan over medium heat. Add 1/2 cup of tomato sauce and simmer for 5 minutes. Remove the eggplant from the oven and top with the tomato sauce. Sprinkle with additional Parmesan cheese and bake for an additional 10 minutes. Serve with cooked whole wheat pasta. Prep time: 20 minutes.

8. Vegetable Stir-Fry: Heat 1 tablespoon of sesame oil in a large skillet over medium-high heat. Add 2 cloves minced garlic, 1/2 teaspoon freshly grated ginger, 1 chopped onion, and 1 chopped red bell pepper. Sauté for 3 minutes. Add 3 cups of chopped vegetables of your choice (such as broccoli, carrots, mushrooms, and snow peas). Cook for an additional 5 minutes until the vegetables are tender. Add 2 tablespoons of reduced-sodium soy sauce and 1 tablespoon of honey and stir until combined. Serve with cooked brown rice. Prep time: 15 minutes.

9. Baked Tofu and Veggies: Preheat oven to 375°F. Line a baking sheet with parchment paper. Cut 1 pound of firm tofu into cubes and place on the baking sheet. Drizzle with 1 tablespoon of olive oil and season with 1 teaspoon of garlic powder, 1 teaspoon of dried oregano, and 1/4 teaspoon of salt. Bake for 15-20 minutes or until the tofu is golden brown. Meanwhile, heat 1 tablespoon of olive oil in a large skillet over medium-high heat. Add 1 chopped onion and 2 cloves minced garlic and sauté for 3 minutes. Add a variety of vegetables of your choice (such as bell peppers, mushrooms, and carrots). Cook for an additional 5 minutes. Add the cooked tofu to the skillet and stir until combined. Serve with cooked brown rice. Prep time: 20 minutes.

10. Baked Halibut with Spinach: Preheat oven to 350°F. Line a baking sheet with parchment paper. Place 2 (4-ounce) halibut filets on the baking sheet and season with 1/4 teaspoon of salt and 1/4 teaspoon of freshly ground black pepper. Bake for 12-15 minutes or until the fish is cooked through. Meanwhile, heat 1 tablespoon of olive oil in a large skillet over medium heat. Add 1 bag of baby spinach and sauté for 3 minutes or until the spinach is wilted. Serve the cooked halibut with the spinach. Prep time: 15 minutes.

11. Grilled Chicken and Avocado Salad: Preheat an outdoor grill or indoor grill pan to medium-high heat. Cut 2 boneless skinless chicken breasts into cubes and season with 1/2 teaspoon of salt and 1/2 teaspoon of freshly ground black pepper. Grill the chicken for 8-10 minutes or until cooked through. Meanwhile, prepare the salad. In a large bowl, combine 2 cups of chopped romaine lettuce, 1 chopped bell pepper, 1/4 cup chopped red onion, 1 avocado, and 1/4 cup crumbled feta cheese. Add the cooked chicken and toss until combined. Drizzle with a simple vinaigrette or your favorite store bought dressing. Prep time: 20 minutes.

12. Baked Salmon and Broccoli: Preheat oven to 375°F. Line a baking sheet with parchment paper. Place 2 (4-ounce) salmon filets on the baking sheet and season with 1/4 teaspoon of salt and 1/4 teaspoon of freshly ground black pepper. Bake for 12-15 minutes or until the salmon is cooked through. Meanwhile, heat 1 tablespoon of olive oil in a large skillet over medium-high heat. Add 1 head of broccoli florets and 1/2 teaspoon of garlic powder. Sauté for 5 minutes or until the broccoli is tender. Serve the salmon and broccoli together. Prep time: 15 minutes.

13. Quinoa Bowl with Roasted Vegetables: Preheat oven to 375°F. Line a baking sheet with parchment paper. Spread 1 cup of cubed sweet potato, 1 cup of cubed butternut squash, 1 cup of sliced mushrooms, and 1 red bell pepper onto the baking sheet. Drizzle with 1 tablespoon of olive oil and season with 1/2 teaspoon of garlic powder, 1/2 teaspoon of dried oregano, and 1/4 teaspoon of salt. Roast for 25-30 minutes or until the vegetables are tender. Meanwhile, bring 1 cup of quinoa and 2 cups of vegetable broth to a boil in a medium saucepan. Reduce the heat and simmer for 15 minutes or until the liquid is absorbed. Fluff with a fork and stir in the roasted vegetables. Serve with freshly chopped parsley, if desired. Prep time: 25 minutes.

14. Grilled Vegetable and Hummus Wraps: Preheat an outdoor grill or indoor grill pan to medium-high heat. Cut a variety of vegetables into large chunks (such as bell peppers, zucchini, mushrooms, and onions). Drizzle with 1 tablespoon of olive oil and season with 1/4 teaspoon of salt and 1/4 teaspoon of freshly ground black pepper. Grill for 8-10 minutes, flipping once halfway through, or until the vegetables are lightly charred and tender. Meanwhile, spread hummus onto 4 whole wheat tortillas. Add the grilled vegetables and wrap up. Slice each wrap in half and serve. Prep time: 15 minutes.

15. Baked Vegetable Frittata: Preheat oven to 375°F. Heat 1 tablespoon of olive oil in a large skillet over medium-high heat. Add 1 chopped onion, 1 chopped red bell pepper, 1 cup of sliced mushrooms, and 1 cup of spinach. Sauté for 5 minutes or until the vegetables are tender. Whisk together 8 eggs, 1/2 cup of milk, 1/2 teaspoon of garlic powder, and 1/4 teaspoon of salt. Pour the egg mixture into the skillet with the vegetables and stir until combined. Bake for 20 minutes or until the frittata is cooked through. Serve with a sprinkle of freshly grated Parmesan cheese, if desired. Prep time: 15 minutes.

16. Chickpea and Kale Salad: In a large bowl, combine 1 can of chickpeas, 1/2 cup of chopped kale, 1/2 cup of chopped bell pepper, 1/4 cup of chopped red onion, and 1/4 cup of crumbled feta cheese. In a small bowl, whisk together 2 tablespoons of olive oil, 1 tablespoon of freshly squeezed lemon juice, 1 teaspoon of Dijon mustard, 1/2 teaspoon of garlic powder, and 1/4 teaspoon of salt. Pour the dressing over the salad and toss until combined. Serve with whole wheat pita chips, if desired. Prep time: 10 minutes.

17. Veggie Pizza: Preheat oven to 375°F. Place a whole wheat pizza crust onto a baking sheet. Spread 1/2 cup of tomato sauce on top of the crust and top with 1/2 cup of shredded mozzarella cheese. Add a variety of vegetables of your choice (such as bell peppers, mushrooms, and onions). Bake for 15-20 minutes or until the cheese is melted and bubbly. Let cool for 5 minutes

Ten (10) Snacks Recipe for Prostate Cancer Prevention

1. Spicy Roasted Chickpeas: Preheat oven to 375F. Drain and rinse 1 can of chickpeas. Place them on a baking sheet and drizzle with 1 tablespoon of olive oil and 1 teaspoon of your favorite spices such as cumin, smoked paprika, garlic powder or chili powder. Bake for 25-30 minutes, stirring occasionally. Enjoy as a crunchy snack or as a topping on salads and soups.

2. Trail Mix: Combine 1/3 cup of nuts, such as walnuts, almonds, or pistachios, 1/3 cup of seeds, such as pumpkin or sunflower, 1/3 cup of dried fruit, such as cranberries or raisins, and 1/4 cup of dark chocolate chips. Place in an airtight container and enjoy as a snack.

3. Hummus and Veggies: Combine 1/2 cup of hummus with 1/2 cup of your favorite diced vegetables, such as bell peppers, cucumbers, carrots, or tomatoes. Serve with whole grain crackers or sliced veggies for a quick and easy snack.

4. Greek Yogurt Parfait: Layer 1/2 cup of Greek yogurt with 1/4 cup of berries or other fruit, such as peaches or pears, and 1 tablespoon of granola. Enjoy as a snack or breakfast.

5. Roasted Edamame: Preheat oven to 400F. Spread 1 cup of shelled edamame on a baking sheet and drizzle with 1 tablespoon of olive oil. Sprinkle with sea salt and any other spices of your choice. Bake for 15 minutes or until lightly golden. Enjoy as a snack or top salads or soups.

6. Avocado Toast: Toast 2 slices of whole grain bread and top each slice with 1/2 an avocado, mashed. Sprinkle with sea salt and freshly ground black pepper to taste. Enjoy as a snack or light meal.

7. Apple and Almond Butter: Slice 1 apple and spread 1 tablespoon of almond butter over each slice. Sprinkle with cinnamon and enjoy as a snack.

8. Baked Sweet Potato Fries: Preheat oven to 400F. Cut 1 sweet potato into thin fries and place on a baking sheet. Drizzle with 1 tablespoon of olive oil and sprinkle with sea salt and any other spices of your choice. Bake for 20-25 minutes, flipping once halfway through. Enjoy as a snack or side dish.

9. Popcorn: Place 1/4 cup of popcorn kernels in a brown paper bag and fold the top. Microwave for 2-3 minutes or until the popping sound slows. Add your favorite seasonings and enjoy as a snack.

10. Protein Smoothie: In a blender, combine 1/2 cup of Greek yogurt, 1/2 cup of milk, 1 scoop of vanilla protein powder, 1/2 cup of frozen fruit, and 1 teaspoon of honey. Blend until smooth and enjoy as a snack.

Ten(10) Desserts Recipes for Prostate Cancer Prevention with prep time and instructions

1. Banana Walnut Muffins – Prep Time: 25 minutes. **Instructions**: Preheat oven to 375°F. Grease 12 muffin cups or line with paper liners. In a medium bowl, mix together 1 cup of whole wheat flour, 1 teaspoon of baking powder, ½ teaspoon of baking soda, and ¼ teaspoon of salt. In a separate bowl, mash 2 ripe bananas and add 1 egg, ½ cup of honey, 1 teaspoon of vanilla extract, and ¼ cup of vegetable oil. Gradually add the wet ingredients to the dry ingredients and stir until just combined. Gently fold in ½ cup of chopped walnuts. Divide the batter evenly among the muffin cups. Bake for 20 minutes or until a toothpick inserted into the center of a muffin comes out clean. Cool for 5 minutes before transferring to a wire rack.

2. Oatmeal Date Cookies – Prep Time: 20 minutes. **Instructions**: Preheat oven to 350°F. In a medium bowl, combine 1 cup of rolled oats, 1 cup of whole wheat flour, ½ teaspoon of baking powder, ¼ teaspoon of baking soda, and ½ teaspoon of ground cinnamon. In a separate bowl, cream together ½ cup of softened butter, ½ cup of honey, and ½ teaspoon of vanilla extract. Gradually add the wet ingredients to the dry ingredients and stir until just combined. Gently fold in 1 cup of chopped dates. Drop the cookie dough onto ungreased baking sheet. Bake for 12 minutes or until golden brown. Cool for 5 minutes before transferring to a wire rack.

3. Apple Crisp – Prep Time: 20 minutes. **Instructions**: Preheat oven to 375°F. Grease an 8-inch baking dish. In a medium bowl, mix together 4 peeled and sliced apples, 1 teaspoon of ground cinnamon, and 1 tablespoon of honey. Spread the mixture evenly in the prepared baking dish. In a separate bowl, mix together 1 cup of rolled oats, ½ cup of whole wheat flour, ¼ cup of chopped walnuts, ¼ cup of honey, and 3 tablespoons of melted butter. Sprinkle the mixture over the apples. Bake for 25 minutes or until the topping is golden brown. Cool for 5 minutes before serving.

4. Blueberry Yogurt Pops – Prep Time: 10 minutes. **Instructions**: Place 1 cup of plain low-fat yogurt, 1 cup of fresh or frozen blueberries, and 1 tablespoon of honey into a blender and blend until smooth. Pour the mixture into ice pop molds and freeze for 2 hours or until firm.

5. Mango Coconut Smoothie – Prep Time: 5 minutes. **Instructions**: Place 1 cup of diced mango, ½ cup of plain low-fat yogurt, ½ cup of coconut milk, and 1 tablespoon of honey into a blender and blend until smooth. Pour the smoothie into a glass and enjoy.

6. Baked Apples – Prep Time: 10 minutes.

Instructions: Preheat oven to 375°F. Grease a 9-inch baking dish. Core 4 apples and place them in the prepared baking dish. In a small bowl, mix together ½ cup of rolled oats, ¼ cup of chopped walnuts, 1 teaspoon of ground cinnamon, and 1 tablespoon of honey. Sprinkle the mixture over the apples. Bake for 25 minutes or until the apples are tender. Cool for 5 minutes before serving.

7. Avocado Chocolate Mousse – Prep Time: 10 minutes.

Instructions: Place 1 ripe avocado, ½ cup of plain low-fat yogurt, 1 teaspoon of vanilla extract, ¼ cup of cocoa powder, and 2 tablespoons of honey into a blender and blend until smooth. Pour the mixture into 4 bowls and refrigerate for 2 hours or until firm.

8. Apple Cinnamon Oatmeal – Prep Time: 10 minutes. **Instructions**: Place 1 cup of rolled oats, 2 diced apples, ½ teaspoon of ground cinnamon, and 2 tablespoons of honey into a saucepan and bring to a boil. Reduce the heat and simmer for 5 minutes or until the oats are tender.

9. Baked Sweet Potato Fries – Prep Time: 10 minutes. **Instructions**: Preheat oven to 375°F. Grease a baking sheet. Cut 2 sweet potatoes into thin strips and place them on the prepared baking sheet. In a small bowl, mix together 1 teaspoon of ground cinnamon, 1 tablespoon of honey, and 1 tablespoon of vegetable oil. Drizzle the mixture over the sweet potatoes and toss to coat. Bake for 20 minutes or until golden brown. Cool for 5 minutes before serving.

10. Berry Crumble – Prep Time: 15 minutes.

Instructions: Preheat oven to 375°F. Grease an 8-inch baking dish. Place 1 cup of raspberries, 1 cup of blueberries, and 1 tablespoon of honey into the prepared baking dish. In a medium bowl, mix together 1 cup of rolled oats, ½ cup of whole wheat flour, ¼ cup of chopped walnuts, and 3 tablespoons of melted butter. Sprinkle the mixture over the berries. Bake for 25 minutes or until the topping is golden brown. Cool for 5 minutes before serving.

CONCLUSION

Among the most prevalent cancers in males is prostate cancer. It is a slow-growing cancer that affects the prostate gland, which is located in the pelvic area and is responsible for producing semen. While there is no single cause of prostate cancer, certain lifestyle and dietary choices can increase the risk of developing this type of cancer.

The Prostate Cancer Cookbook is a great resource for men and their families who are looking to make lifestyle and diet changes that may reduce their risk of developing prostate cancer. The book offers a wide range of recipes that are both healthy and flavorful, with an emphasis on fresh, whole foods. It also includes information about nutrition and the importance of a balanced diet and the benefits of physical activity. Additionally, the book provides helpful tips and advice on how to make healthy lifestyle changes that can help reduce the risk of prostate cancer.

The Prostate Cancer Cookbook is an invaluable resource for anyone looking to make healthy changes to their lifestyle and diet. It provides a wealth of information and recipes that are easy to follow and understand. Not only does this book provide helpful information and delicious recipes, but it also offers a sense of hope and empowerment to those who are dealing with prostate cancer.

In conclusion, the Prostate Cancer Cookbook is an invaluable resource for anyone looking to make healthy changes to their lifestyle and diet. It provides a wealth of information and recipes that are easy to follow and understand. Additionally, it offers a sense of hope and empowerment to those who are dealing with prostate cancer.

The book is a great way to help reduce the risk of prostate cancer and improve overall health and wellbeing.

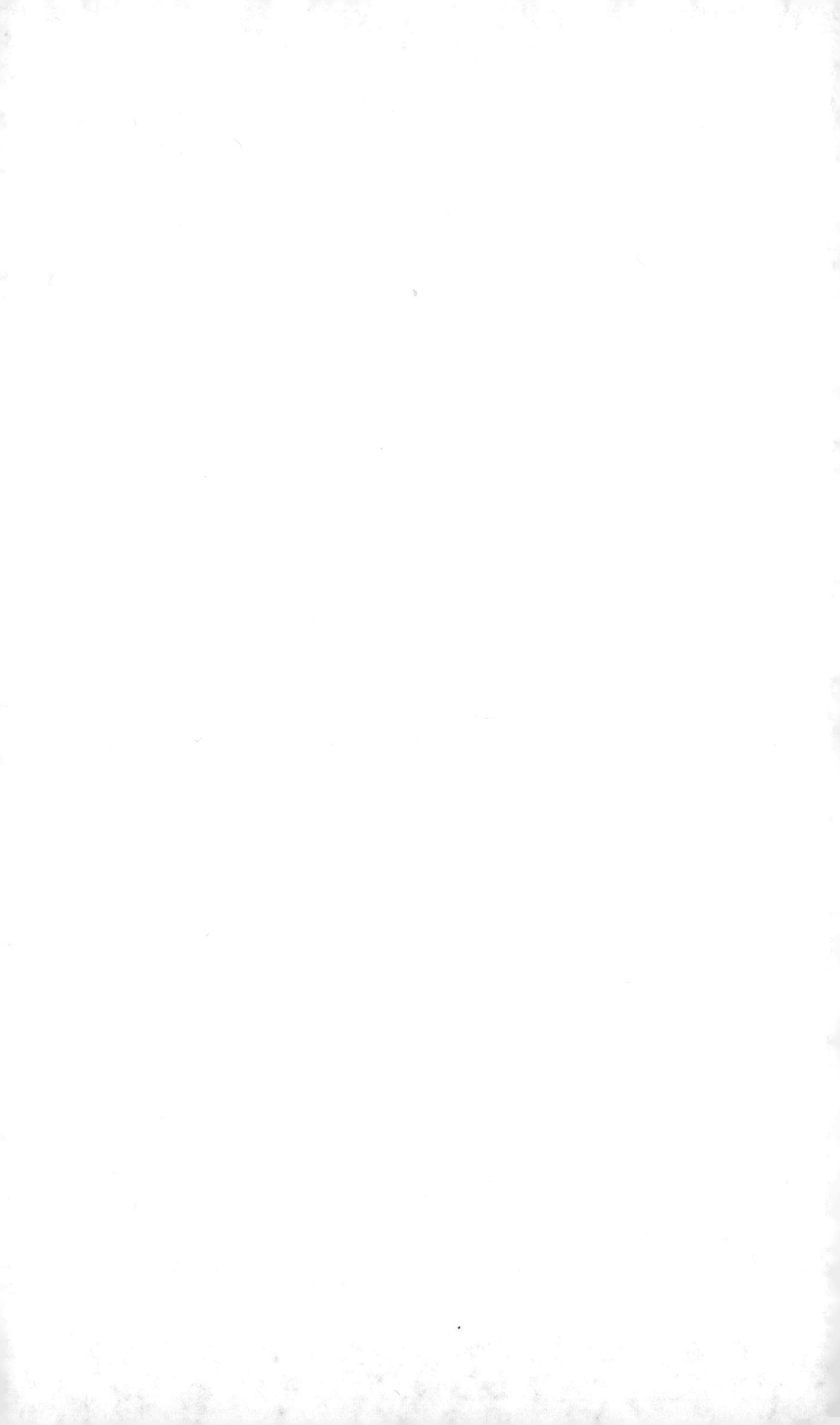